ANGIOPLASTY & STENTS

FOR NARROWED ARTERIES AND VEIN BYPASS GRAFTS

by **Julia Ann Purcell, RN, MN, FAAN**

Clinical Nursing Specialist, Cardiology

1968-1996

This book is not to be used to replace any of your doctor's advice or treatment. It is to help you understand more about angioplasty.

What is angioplasty?

Angioplasty is a **procedure** used **to open clogged arteries or vein bypass grafts.** When angioplasty works well to open an artery, blood flow is improved. Often a small coil (**stent**) is left in the newly opened artery to help keep it open over time. Angioplasty is **not surgery**, and you will be awake while it is being done. Some people go home the day of the procedure and others stay in the hospital at least one night.

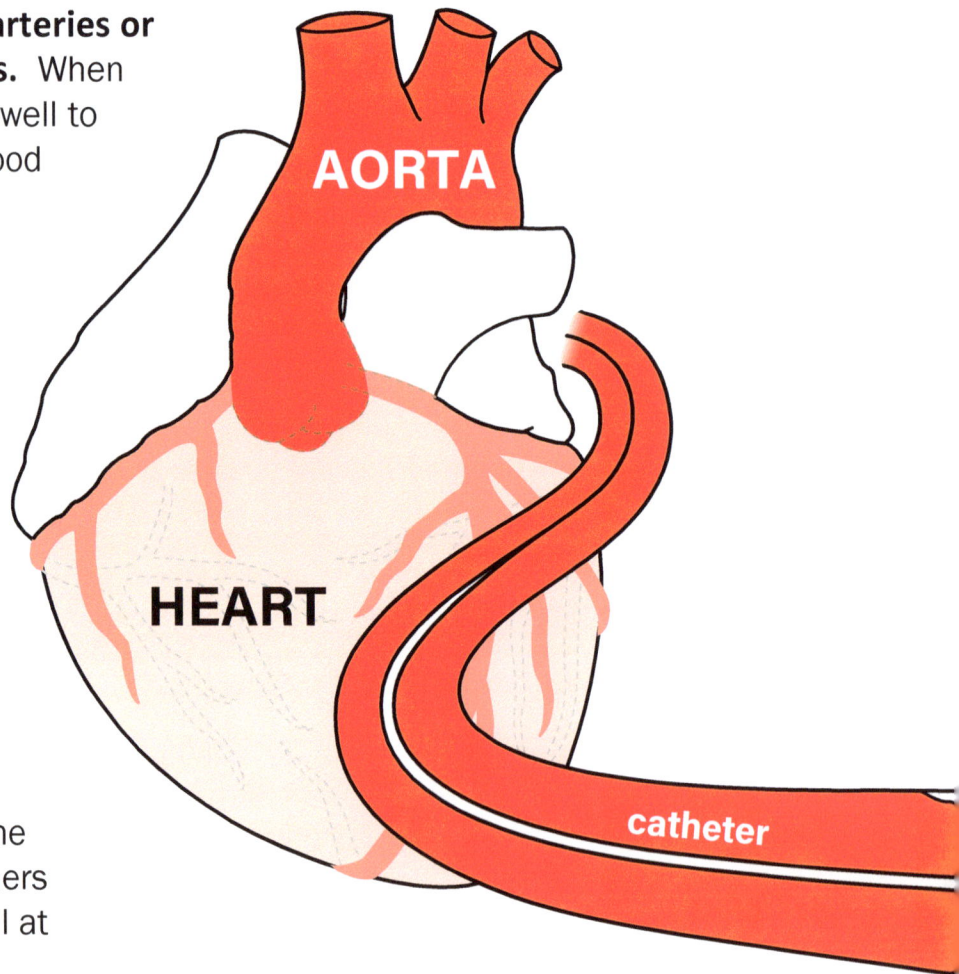

AORTA

HEART

catheter

Angioplasty is only a treatment to open clogged arteries or vein bypass grafts. Most people need to make healthier lifestyle changes and take a drug (often a 'statin') to control blood fats and avoid new fatty buildup (plaque). Measures to keep existing fatty plaque 'stable' are also needed. When the inner lining on a fatty buildup tears (plaque rupture), a blood clot forms to seal it. If big enough, the clot can stop blood flow through that artery. Studies show daily low-dose aspirin and/or an antiplatelet drug along with a 'statin' help keep fatty plaque stable.

Angioplasty and/or stent placement can be done in many body arteries (or vein bypass grafts). In this book, the symbols below will help you know when the angioplasty involves arteries in the heart, kidney, arm, leg or other body arteries (for example, head and neck arteries):

heart
(often called PTCA or PCI - percutaneous coronary intervention*)

kidney
(often called renal angioplasty*)

leg, arm, neck or other body artery
(called [artery name] angioplasty*)

*Definitions:

percutaneous - through the skin

artery name - coronary (heart); renal (kidney); etc

angioplasty - remodeling of a blood vessel

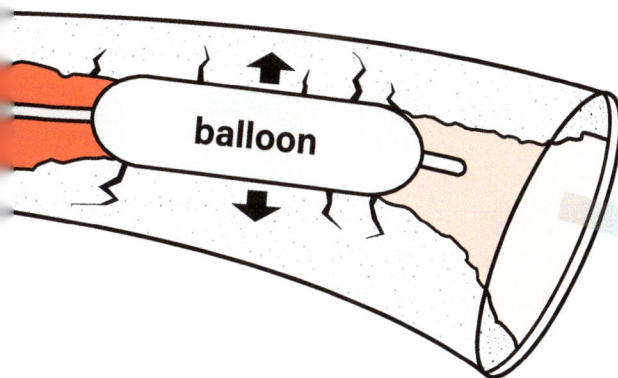

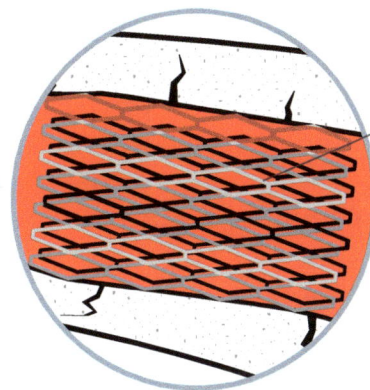

balloon

stent in place after angioplasty

Read these sections to find out more

Buildup in the arteries (atherosclerosis)

The body arteries are like tubes with elastic walls. They carry oxygen-rich blood from the heart to all parts of the body, including the heart muscle itself. Many factors can lead to damage of an artery wall. When certain blood fats are high, it is easier for the fat to build up in the damaged wall. Fatty buildup is more likely when a person:

- smokes

- has a diet high in cholesterol and saturated fat

- has high blood pressure

- doesn't exercise

- is overweight

- has diabetes

- is related to someone who has angina or had a heart attack at an early age

- has a lot of stress and tension

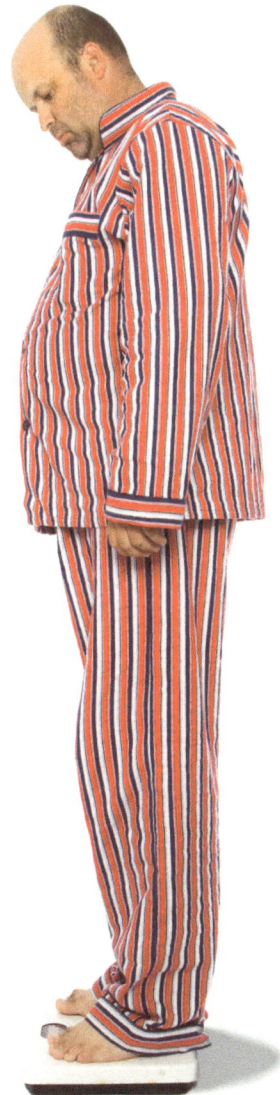

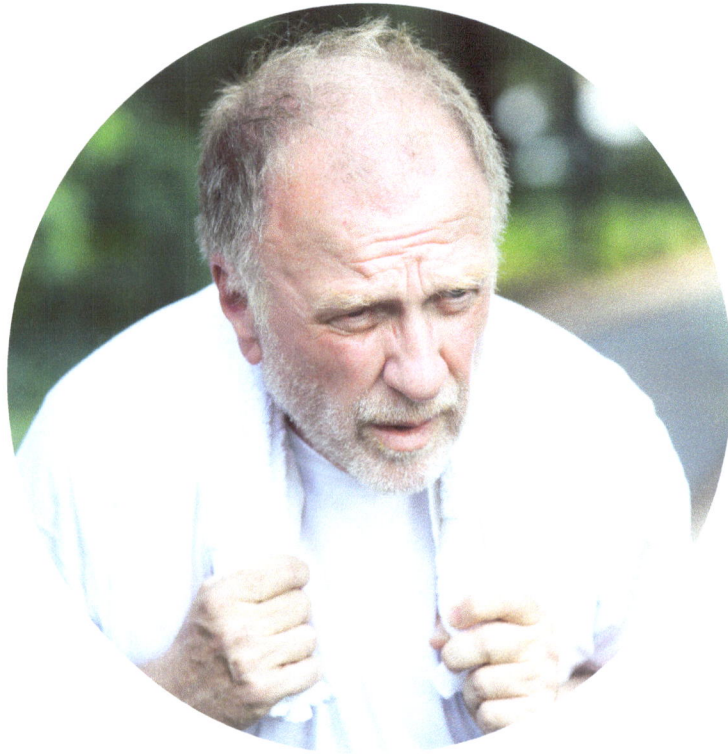

Fatty buildup is much like when rust clogs up a pipe and only a trickle of water can get through. When blood flow is blocked by fatty narrowing, symptoms are likely.

A narrowed heart artery can cause angina (tightness, pressure, squeezing, burning, pain or aching in the chest or either arm; indigestion; discomfort in the upper back; breathlessness, choking, weakness or sweating). Heart damage is likely if a blood clot forms in the tiny channel unless it is opened in time by angioplasty or an intravenous clot-buster.

Blockage in a kidney artery often causes high blood pressure, though you may not know it. (But most high blood pressure is not due to this.) High blood pressure can weaken kidney function and cause them to fail.

Fatty buildup in a leg or arm artery causes pain, cramping or fatigue when you use the limb. Leg artery symptoms are common if you walk a long distance or up a hill.

Warning signs of a narrowed neck artery can include sudden weakness or problems with vision or speech. These are often called "TIA's" (transient ischemic attacks) and relate to which part of the brain the narrowed artery feeds.

Treating fatty buildup

When blockage from fatty buildup is severe, angioplasty is often done to try and improve blood flow. Your doctors may use one or more of these during your angioplasty procedure:

- **Balloon catheters** – inflate and compress the fatty buildup

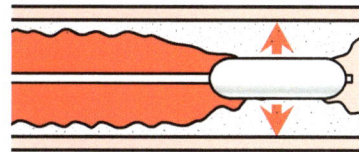

- **Stents** – prop open an artery

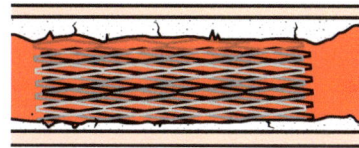

- **Rotational atherectomy catheters** – remove the fatty buildup

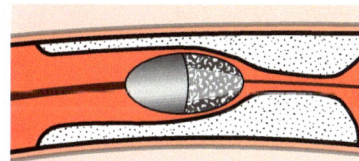

Other catheters may also be needed to:

- take a closer look at a fatty blockage (ultrasound or OCT [optical coherence tomography])

- suck out or prevent blood clots or fatty material from going downstream

- see how much a blockage is changing blood flow

- maintain blood flow through a blocked artery during the procedure

balloon angioplasty

With balloon angioplasty, a catheter (thin, flexible tube) with a balloon on the end is placed in the clogged artery. The balloon is inflated and deflated a number of times to stretch the narrowed opening and compress the fatty buildup.

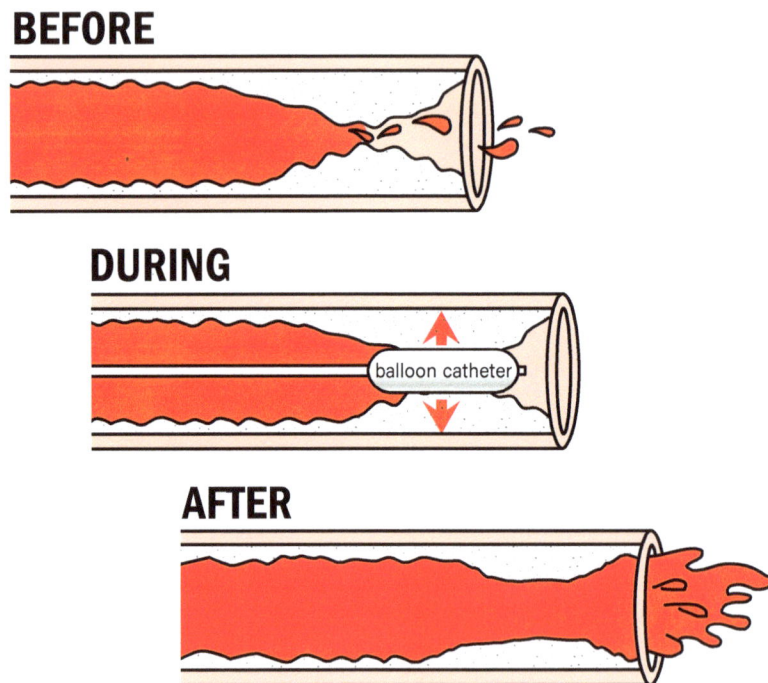

BEFORE

DURING

balloon catheter

AFTER

Some balloon catheters have a cutting device to make small cuts in the fatty buildup as the balloon is expanding. These cuts in the fat make it easier for the balloon to expand and put less stress on the artery wall.

Some leg artery balloon catheters are coated with a drug which is released during angioplasty to discourage more artery narrowing.

stents

Angioplasty often includes placement of one or more pieces of stainless steel mesh (called stents) in the narrowed artery. Stents help prop an artery open to allow better blood flow.

A stent comes tightly wound on a tiny balloon catheter. Once the catheter is guided to the site, the balloon is inflated to expand the stent.

After the balloon catheter is removed, X-ray or ultrasound pictures are made to make sure the stent is fully expanded. Once a stent is fully expanded, it is left in place to prop the artery open and allow better blood flow.

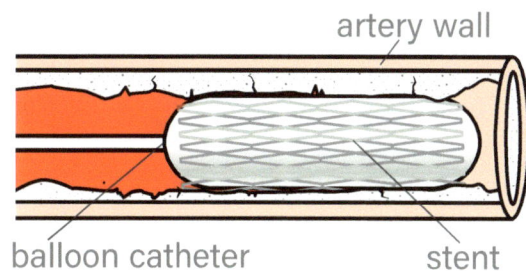

artery wall

balloon catheter   stent

balloon catheter expanding stent in place

Your doctor will choose whether a bare metal stent (BMS) or a drug-eluting stent (DES) is best for your blocked artery. Since blood clots can form in both, anti-clotting drugs are needed for weeks, months or even years. Bare metal stents may need anti-clotting drugs for less

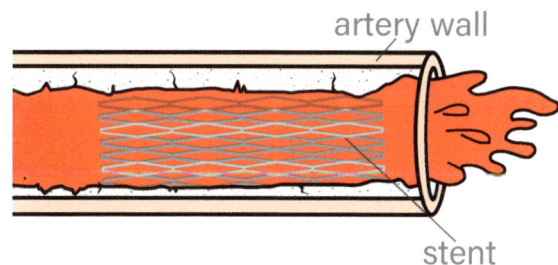

artery wall

stent

time. A DES slowly releases a drug to discourage smooth muscle cell buildup in the dilated artery. This buildup (restenosis) blocks blood flow just like the fatty blockage. Most of today's stents are metal so tell your doctor if you have stainless steel or nickel allergy.

Newer DES stents are partially or fully absorbable. The Boston Scientific Synergy™ DES has a polymer coating which goes away in 3-4 months. Abbott makes a fully absorbable "stent" called the Absorb GT1™ vascular scaffold. It takes about 3 years to absorb. Absorbable stents help an artery wall regain a more flexible shape.

atherectomy

When fatty buildup needs to be removed during angioplasty, an atherectomy catheter is used. The **rotational atherectomy catheter** is a rotary burr covered with tiny diamonds. It turns very fast to grind away buildup into tiny bits your body can absorb.

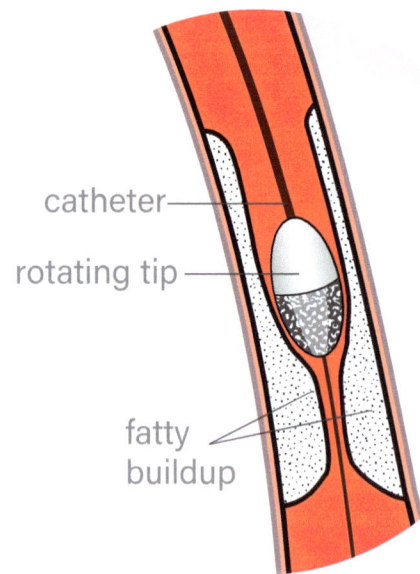

rotational atherectomy catheter (Rotablator®)

other catheters

Before opening the narrowed artery, your doctor may insert:

- a catheter for intravascular ultrasound (IVUS) or use optical coherence tomography (OCT) to take a closer look at the fatty blockage

and/or

- a guidewire through the blockage to measure blood flow (fractional flow reserve or FFR)

These often help in making the decision if, when or how an artery should be opened and which stent (if any) would work best.

Sometimes an 'extraction' catheter is used before angioplasty to suck out blood clots inside the narrowed artery. Once the clot is removed, balloon angioplasty and/or stenting can be done.

A catheter to keep blood clots (or fatty material) from going downstream is usually needed during angioplasty in the neck/head arteries and with vein bypass grafts. Your doctor may call the catheter a 'filter' or an EPD (embolic protection device). Examples include:

- SpiderFX™

- FilterWire EZ™

- Angioguard®

- Guardwire®

- Emboshield®

- Rubicon filter®

- RX Accunet®

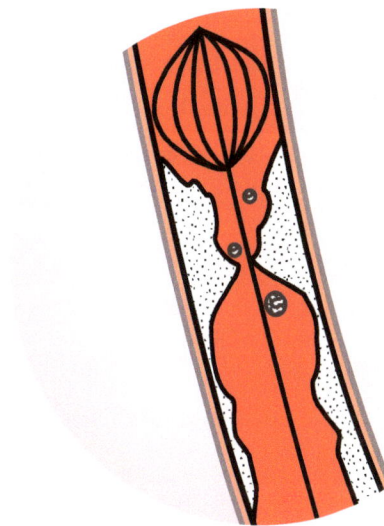

Angioguard®

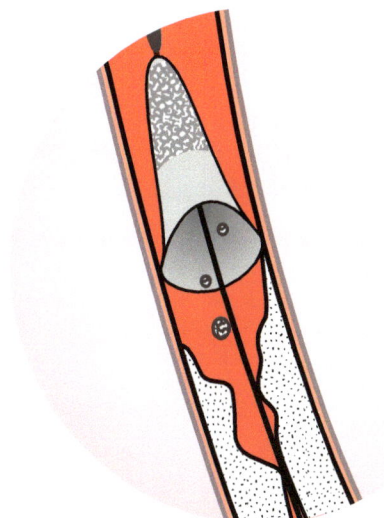

FilterWire EZ™

radiation (brachytherapy) and in-stent restenosis

Heart arteries opened with angioplasty can get blocked again by rapid growth of smooth muscle cells at the site (restenosis). Although restenosis is likely part of your body's effort to heal after angioplasty, the buildup can block blood flow and cause more symptoms. Using a catheter to deliver radiation inside an artery or stent is called brachytherapy.

Restenosis is more likely inside a bare metal stent. Drug-eluting stents (DES) help prevent early buildup of smooth muscle cells inside a stent. If the inside of a bare metal stent gets a buildup of smooth muscle cells, your doctor may choose to replace it with a drug-eluting stent or do brachytherapy.

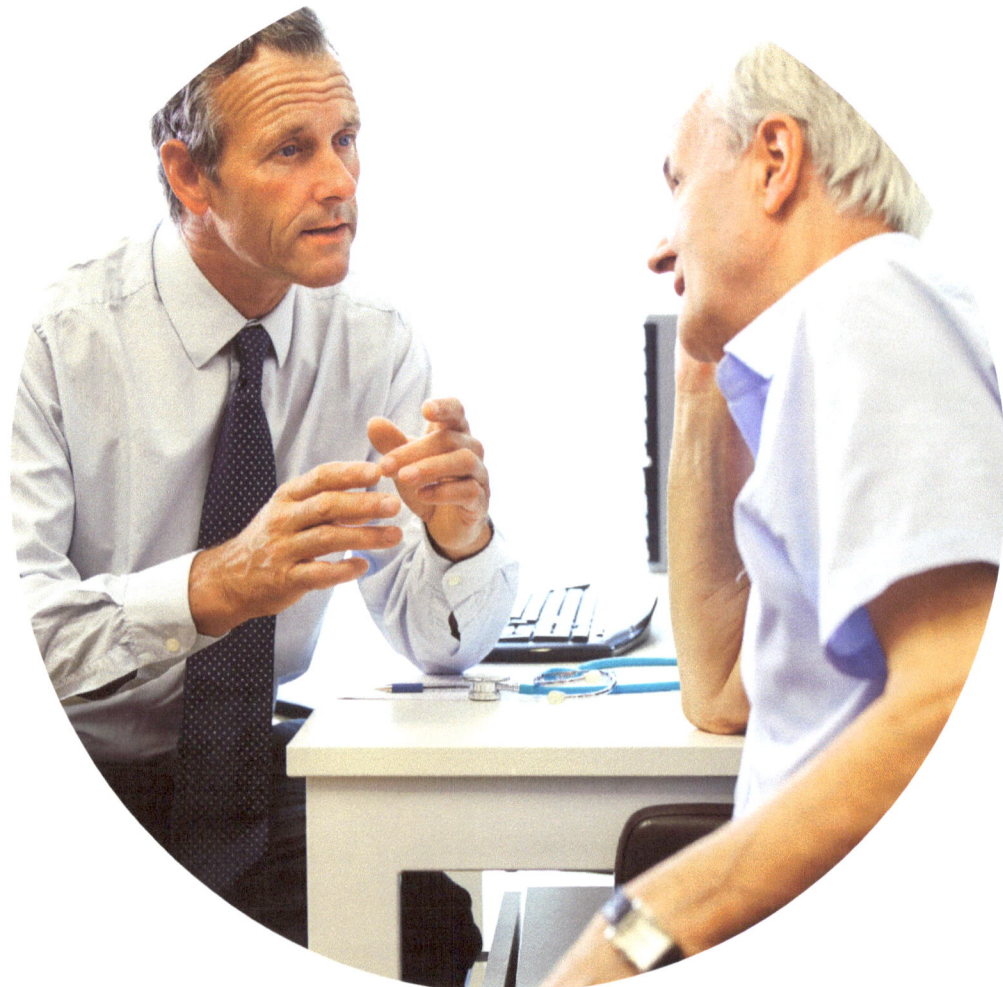

Preventing clots

Persons **not** taking daily aspirin at home are often given a full-size, non-coated aspirin before angioplasty in a heart artery. IV (intravenous) anti-clotting drugs are often used during angioplasty and sometimes for a few hours afterward to prevent blood clots. Anti-clotting drugs, like Heparin, Angiomax®, Arixtra® or argatroban are common choices.

Often anti-clotting therapy continues at home with a drug to discourage the blood platelets from clumping and starting a clot. Anti-platelet drugs include a 75 or 80 mg daily dose of aspirin and/or one of these: Plavix® (clopidogrel); Effient® (prasugrel) or Brilinta® (ticagrelor). Sometimes an oral anticoagulant is used instead. Examples include Coumadin®, Pradaxa®, Eliquis® or Xarelto®. **An anti-clotting drug(s) is crucial to prevent blood clots inside a newly placed stent(s).**

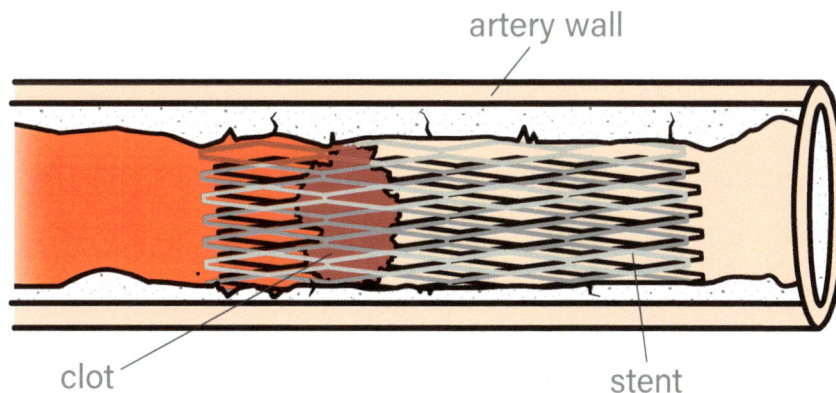

artery wall

clot

stent

Not taking your anti-clotting drugs can lead to sudden clotting inside the stent and heart attack. This can be life-threatening.

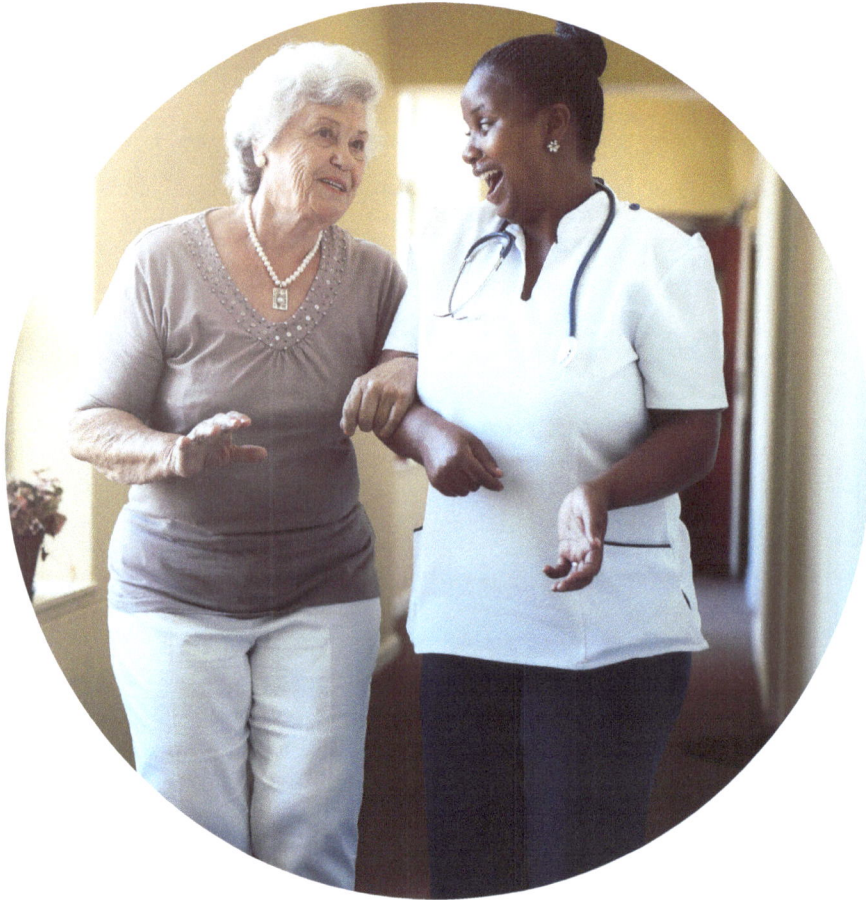

These are highlights of anti-clotting therapy after angioplasty:

- **DO NOT leave the hospital without a prescription for the anti-clotting drug(s) your doctor has ordered for you.**

- **Although blood tests aren't routine when taking aspirin, an anti-platelet drug, or an anticoagulant like apixaban (Eliquis®), dabigatran (Pradaxa®) or rivaroxaban (Xarelto®), always call your doctor right away if you have unusual bleeding or bruising.**

- **NEVER stop anti-clotting drugs on your own. Don't miss a dose or take any extra. When a stent(s) is placed during angioplasty, anti-clotting therapy is crucial for weeks, months or even years.**

- **If you are having surgery or any invasive procedure, consult your heart doctor about what to do about your anti-clotting drug(s).**

Getting ready for angioplasty

Most people having angioplasty are told not to eat or drink anything after midnight the night before the procedure. Often a drug to control cholesterol (statin) is given before your procedure. Those having kidney (renal) angioplasty may be asked not to eat solid foods but to drink a lot of liquids. A nurse will tell you what your doctor has ordered.

You will talk with a doctor or other member of the healthcare team about your symptoms and have a brief physical exam. He or she will explain the risks of the procedure and ask you to sign a consent form.

The consent form will list the risks of angioplasty. These include risks common to any x-ray procedure through a blood vessel (bleeding or swelling at the puncture site; rarely a heart attack or stroke). Spasm, blockage or a tear can also occur in the artery being opened. These can happen during, or shortly after angioplasty. Your doctor will review the risks with you, as well as any emergency treatment that might be needed. Although angioplasty has a high success rate, life-threatening complications can occur.

Take with you to the hospital:

- **a list of all of your medicines —** or the bottles (Take your medicines as usual until your doctor or nurse tells you not to.)

- any **recent ECG's** or **blood test reports** (This may prevent repeating the tests.)

Tell your doctor if you have:

- allergy to iodine, x-ray dye, shellfish or other medicines

- a bleeding history or problems taking aspirin or anti-clotting drugs

- back pain or problems using a urinal or bedpan while lying on your back

Any hair will be removed around the artery where the angioplasty catheter will be put in, and the site will be cleaned with a special soap. A needle is put into an arm vein and attached with tubing to IV (intravenous) fluids. Medicines and fluids can then be given through the tubing.

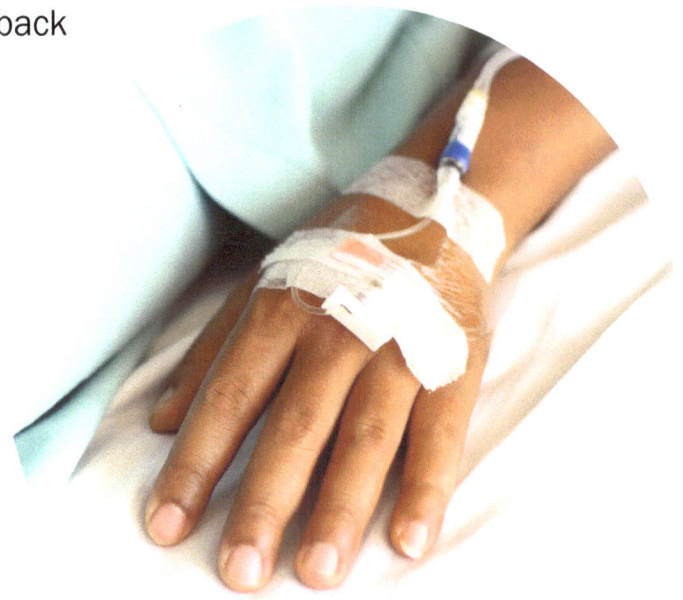

You will most likely be awake during the procedure. Medicine will be given to help you relax either before you leave your room or after you are in the x-ray suite. Expect to feel drowsy — perhaps even a little dizzy. Some people fall asleep during this time. Others are awake but don't recall the procedure. It's rare, but the relaxing medicine can also cause itching or nausea.

catheter insertion

Once you are in the x-ray suite, ECG pads (electrodes) are placed on your arms, legs and/or trunk. These record your heartbeat. Your blood pressure is also checked from time to time or monitored through the catheter.

The shaved site is scrubbed with a special soap, and a numbing medicine is injected under the skin. You will be draped with a sterile sheet and asked to keep your hands under it. An introducer sheath (tube) is put into either the groin, wrist or elbow artery. A catheter is guided through this sheath to the narrowed artery.

X-ray dye ("contrast") is put in to help see any artery narrowings or blockage. (The dye may cause a "hot" feeling or brief nausea.) You will see picture images on the monitor as the camera moves around you.

Catheter entering groin artery

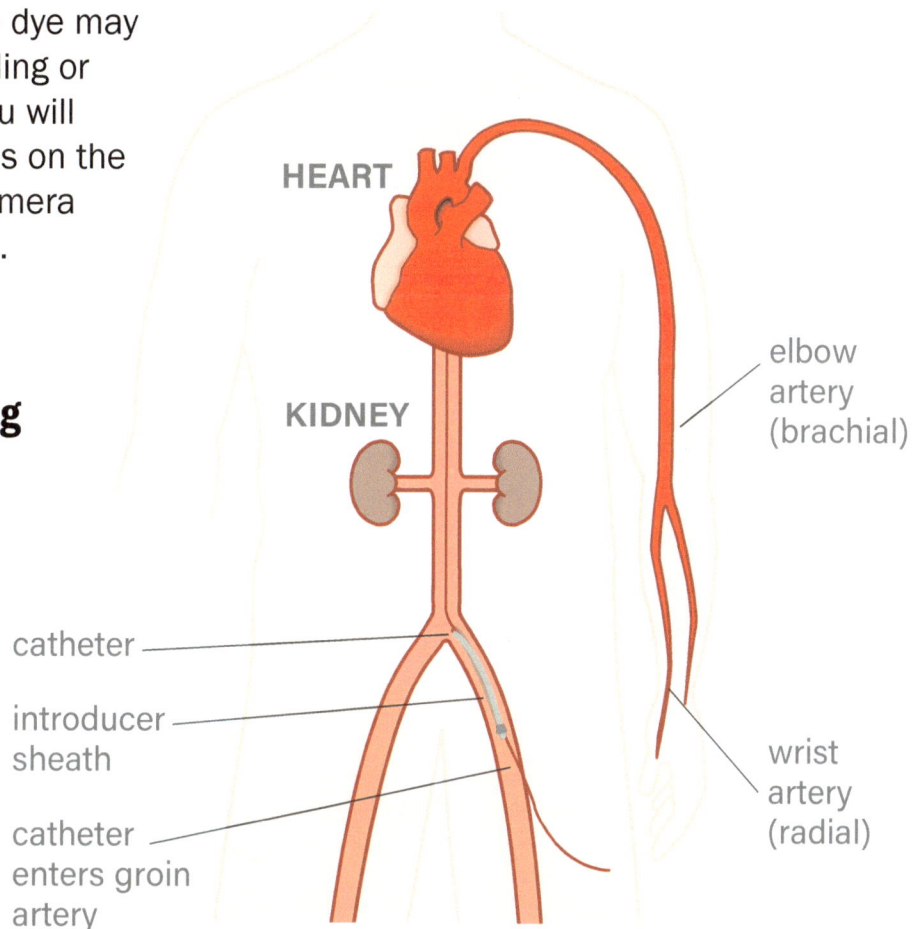

HEART

KIDNEY

elbow artery (brachial)

wrist artery (radial)

catheter

introducer sheath

catheter enters groin artery

The angioplasty

As the doctor puts the angioplasty catheter in a narrowed heart artery, you may be asked to cough or take a deep breath. This helps clear the x-ray dye from the artery and improve the quality of the pictures.

When the catheter is in place, the doctor will closely watch the x-ray view of the artery. You may have your original symptoms for a few moments during the procedure. This happens because the inflated balloon or catheter stops blood flow through the narrowed artery for a short time. Though these symptoms are fairly common, tell the doctor so that he or she can deflate the balloon or give medicines to help the pain.

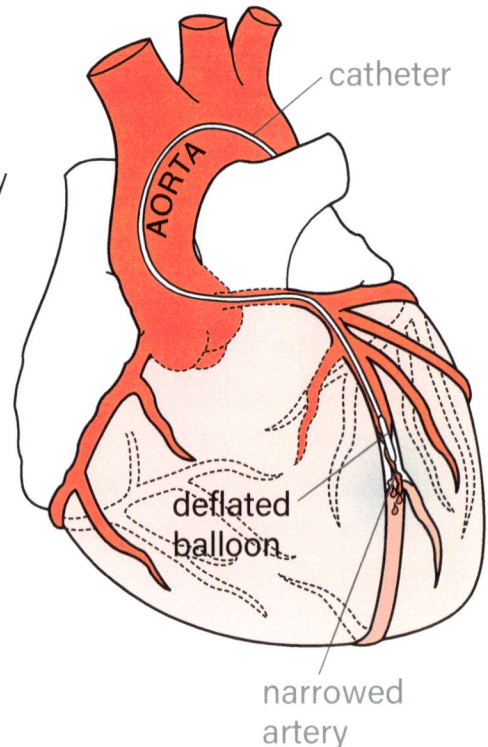

catheter

AORTA

deflated balloon

narrowed artery

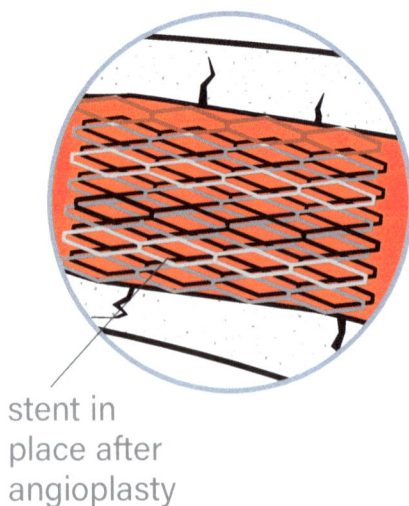

stent in place after angioplasty

Balloon angioplasty often takes several balloon inflations to flatten the fatty buildup. After the artery has been opened, the catheter is removed. X-ray dye is then injected into the narrowed artery to see if the inside opening is big enough. A stent (or scaffold) may be left in place to help keep the artery open.

After angioplasty

What happens right after angioplasty will depend on whether you had angioplasty in a heart, kidney, arm, leg or other body artery.

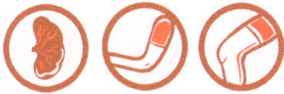

for patients having angioplasty in any artery not involving the heart

Angioplasty in a kidney, arm or leg artery is usually a same day procedure. Pressure will be applied to the puncture site for 20 to 30 minutes. A bandage is put on, and several hours of bedrest begin. During this time, **you must not bend the site where the catheter was put in.** A nurse will check your vital signs (heart rate, blood pressure, etc.) and pulses. Most of the time, solid food and liquids are allowed right away. Most patients go home the same day.

Special precautions are needed when angioplasty is done on a narrowed neck or head artery. Ask your doctor for information about head and neck artery angioplasty and stents.

Keep your head and shoulders on the pillow to avoid bending your knee or hip.

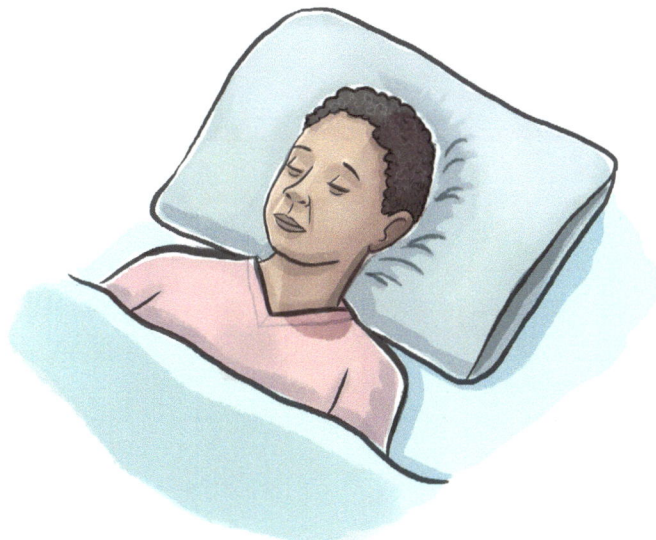

for patients having heart artery angioplasty

Some patients having heart angioplasty return home on the same day but others stay in the hospital for one night. Nurses monitor your heart and site recovery along with giving medicines. Recovery after heart angioplasty varies with the puncture site (leg, wrist or elbow) and how the artery is sealed. It may also vary with the type and amount of anti-clotting drugs used.

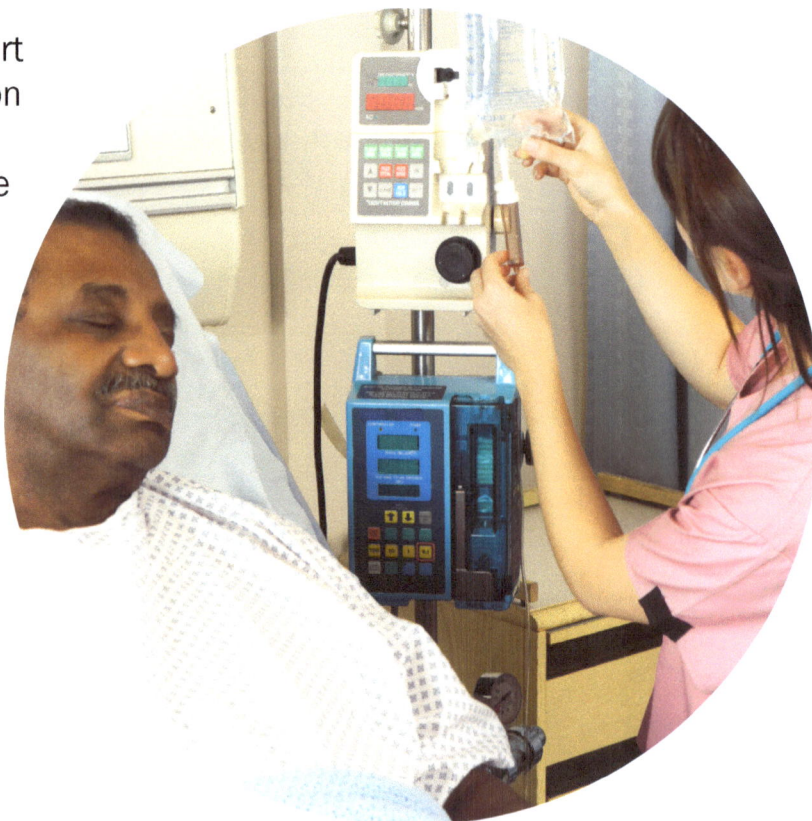

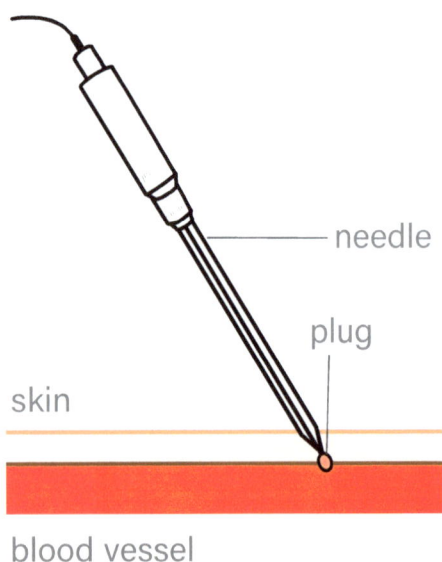

needle

plug

skin

blood vessel

Recovery: leg puncture site

Heart angioplasty is often done through a sheath in a large upper leg (groin) artery. Since at least one IV drug is given to prevent clots, care is needed to prevent bleeding as the sheath is taken out. At the end of the procedure, a patch or plug made of thrombin, collagen or other material may be used to seal the artery. At other times, a device that places absorbable stitches inside the artery can be used.

sheath removal

Several hours of bed rest are needed before the leg angioplasty sheath is removed. This is so the blood can return to normal clotting. As the sheath is removed, a plastic pressure strap is often placed over the puncture site.

After blood checks show good clotting times, the sheath can be removed. Firm hand pressure must then be applied or a pressure clamp placed on the puncture site. Then a bandage is applied and left overnight on the site.

Firm pressure with a Femostop® (or 2–3 fingers) is needed to stop bleeding at the puncture site when absorbable sutures (stitches), a patch or plug are **not** used to seal the artery.

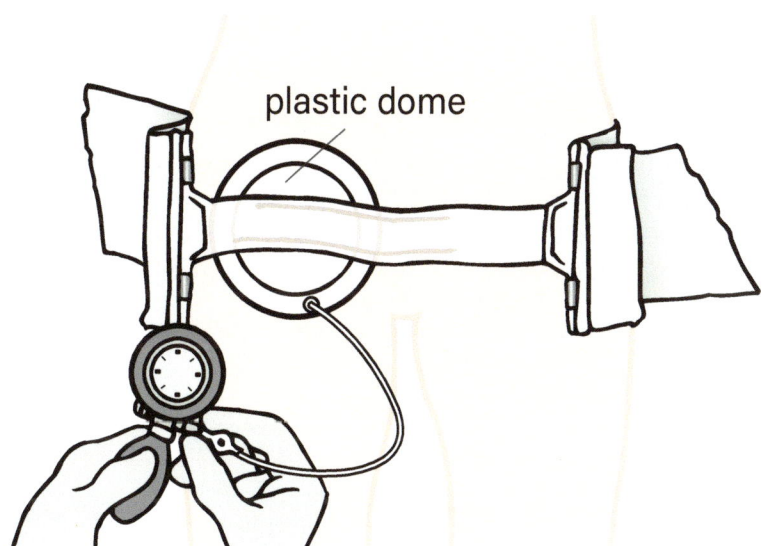

plastic dome

bedrest

Most angioplasty patients with a leg artery puncture site need several hours of bed rest after the sheath is removed. A few extra hours may be needed when heparin or other anti-clotting drugs are used. When a leg artery puncture is closed with stitches or certain plugs, walking may be allowed within a few hours of the procedure.

reminders for leg puncture site recovery

Let the nurse know if you feel any wetness, warmth, swelling or pain at the site. This may mean you are bleeding. You will be reminded **NOT to bend the knee** of the affected leg. You don't need to hold this leg stiff. Just keep it straight. Wiggling your ankle or toes from time to time may help you stay comfortable. Having pressure on the puncture site and keeping it straight are very important to prevent bleeding. If you cough, sneeze or laugh hard while resting, hold firm pressure over the bandage. If you feel like you may vomit, DO NOT SIT UP! Turn to the side of the bed, and keep the bandaged leg straight.

no sitting

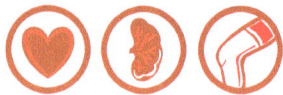

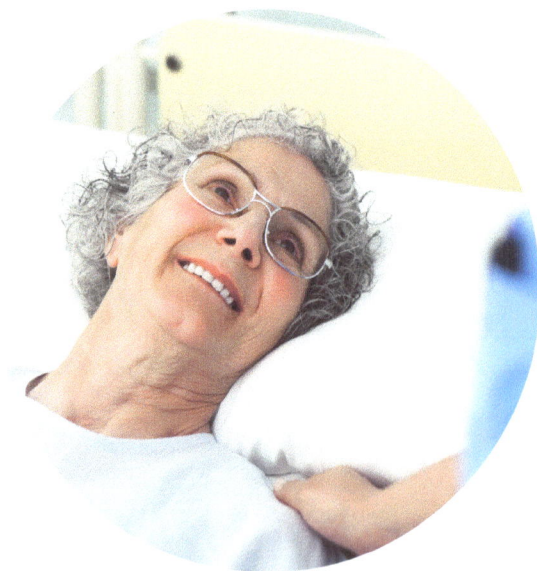

Some back or leg pain is likely from having to lie still. Ask your nurse for pain medicine before your pain gets too bad. Bend your other leg from time to time for relief. **Do not** lift your head off the pillow. Doing this will cause muscles to tighten near the puncture site and may affect the artery seal. If you have trouble using a urinal or bedpan while lying on your back, tell the nurse. **Do not get out of bed!** When you are able to get out of bed for the first time, the nurse will check your blood pressure to make sure there is no problem with bleeding or dizziness.

Recovery: elbow or wrist puncture site (less commonly used)

Wrist (radial) arteries are being used more often in the US for angioplasty. Sometimes the elbow (brachial) artery is used instead. As the sheath is removed from a wrist artery, a plastic pressure strap is often placed over the puncture site and the arm or hand is raised up on 1-2 pillows. The pulses and blood flow in the hand will be checked often. A syringe attached to the air port can vary the pressure under the plastic strap as needed. If your hand or arm turns blue or gets painful and cold to the touch, tell your nurse or doctor right away.

Most people can get out of bed within a few hours and often go home on the same day. A handboard (or sling) to prevent bending near the puncture site may be used. Your doctor may ask you to avoid intense arm or wrist activity for a period of time. This may include **not** using a computer or writing for a few days.

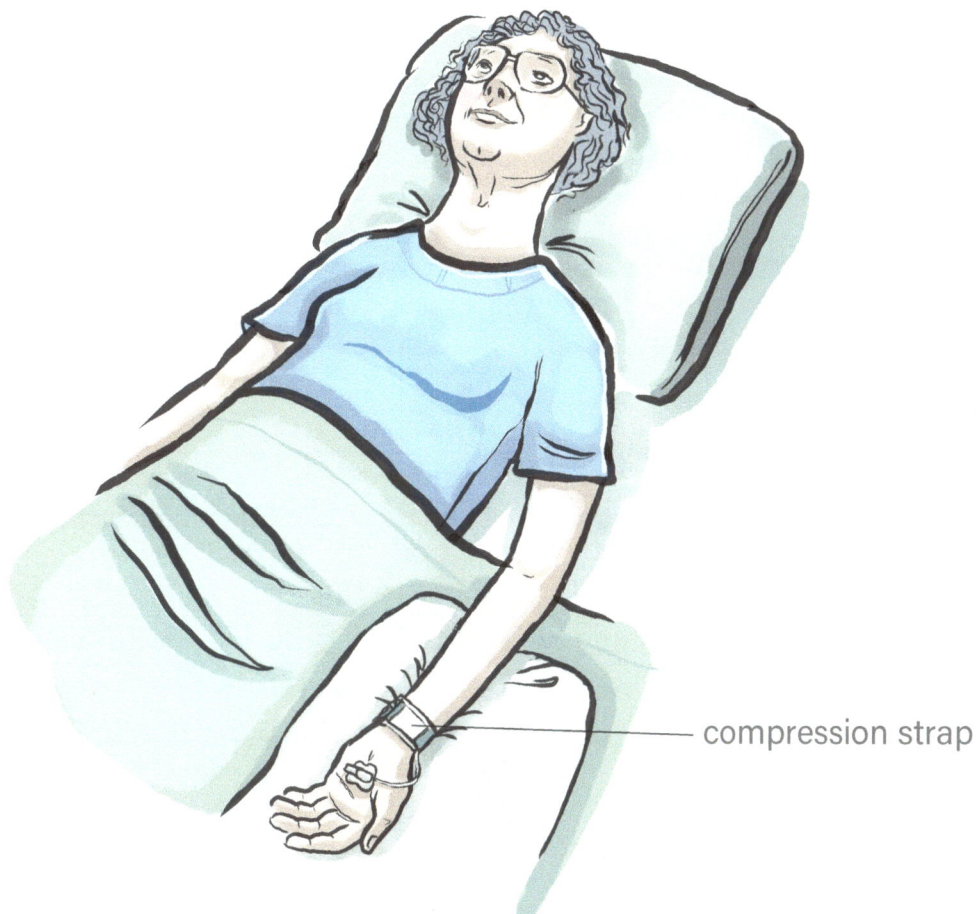

compression strap

CAUTION

Let your nurse know right away if you notice **any** of these at the puncture site:

- a wet, warm feeling

- sharp or burning pain

- swelling near the site

Any of these may mean that the puncture site is bleeding. Also, call the nurse right away if you have nausea, chest pain or any of the other symptoms that caused you to see your doctor. If severe or prolonged chest pain does occur after heart angioplasty, a second angioplasty or bypass surgery may be needed.

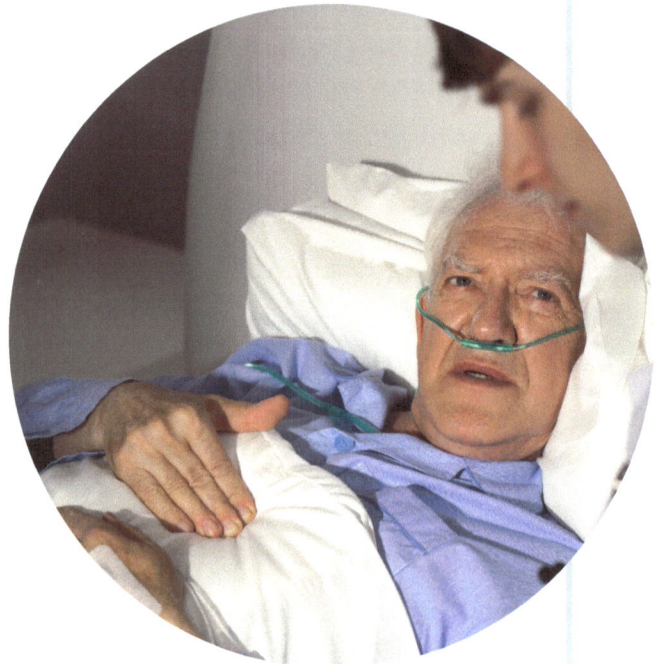

You may have to urinate often as your body gets rid of the dye used during angioplasty. This fluid needs to be replaced by IV fluids and liquids you drink. Since vomiting can occur after heart angioplasty, only liquids may be offered during the first few hours. Solid foods are OK after the sheath is removed. If you are diabetic, your insulin may be held, delayed or the dosage reduced on the day of angioplasty.

Going home

A Band-Aid® or smaller dressing replaces the original bandage. As you change the Band-Aid® each day, check for any new swelling or signs of infection (new discomfort, redness, hot areas or drainage). A bruise at the site as well as soreness and a few days of fatigue are common. Most people can take a shower in 24 to 48 hours. Ask your doctor when it is OK for you. Avoid tub baths for 5-7 days to prevent infection.

Unless there was a recent heart damage, most people return to their normal routine within a few days after angioplasty. Some doctors advise that you not jog or lift things that weigh more than 10 lbs in the first few days after you go home. If you had a groin procedure, break up long sitting times by walking around. People who have a groin lump after angioplasty or take an anti-clotting drug(s) are often told to delay things like tennis and running. Check with your doctor about this, especially if a plug was used to seal the artery/puncture site.

Take a walking break.

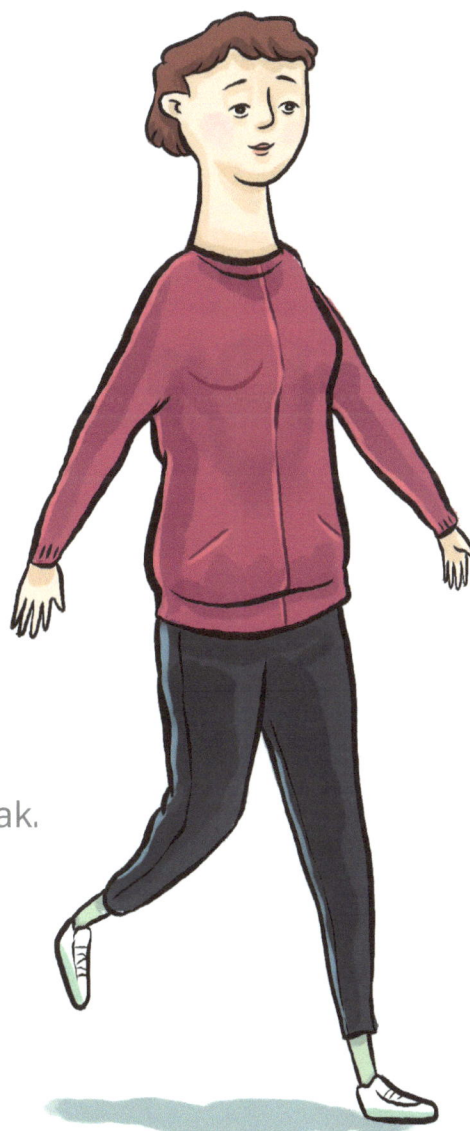

Successful angioplasty for most people means:

heart (coronary)
fewer or no symptoms of angina or shortness of breath.

kidney (renal)
high blood pressure may go down over time and the risk of kidney failure may be reduced. (Note: Follow-up checks of blood pressure are done so that medicines can be reduced— or stopped.)

arm, leg or other body artery
less severe or no pain/cramps or other symptoms of impaired blood flow.

How much relief you get depends on how much the artery can be opened, as well as how many other arteries remain blocked. After your angioplasty, be sure to let your doctor know if you are having any more symptoms.

Since the success with angioplasty varies, ask your doctor about:

- the amount of improvement in the artery opening

- how likely it is that your symptoms will return

- medicines and activity limits (if any)

- changes in lifestyle needed to reduce the risk of more fatty buildup

- follow-up office visits and tests

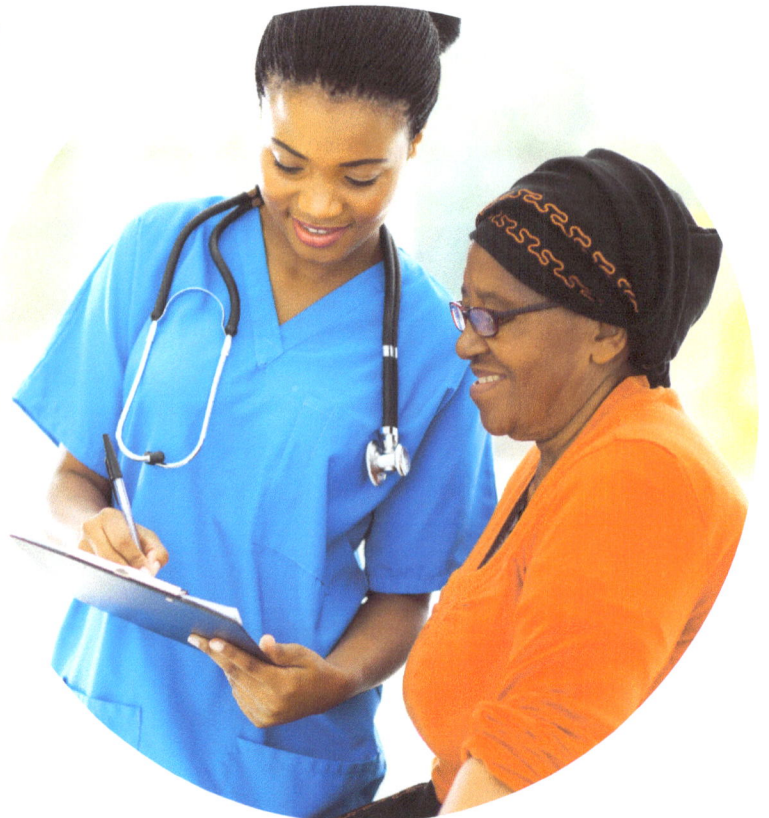

Preventing fatty buildup

Once an artery has been opened, you may feel "cured" and ready to return to old habits. **But angioplasty is a treatment for fatty buildup, not a cure.** Taking daily, low-dose aspirin and a drug to control blood fats, along with healthy lifestyle changes can help keep your fatty plaque stable. It can also help prevent future fat buildup. Many people find cardiac rehab very helpful in learning to live heart-healthy.

quit smoking

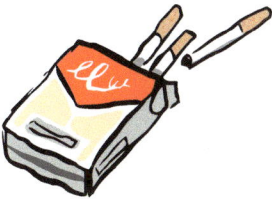

Smoking raises the risks of high blood pressure, heart attack, stroke, cancer and death. It also makes it easier for the blood to clot. Quitting is one of the best things you can do to reduce chances of more blockage. If you have trouble quitting, ask your doctor if medicine would be an option for you.

control blood fats

Total cholesterol should be less than 200 mg/dL.* The good cholesterol (HDL) should be **over** 40 mg/dL in men and 50 mg/dL in women. The bad cholesterol (LDL) should be **less than** 100 mg/dL. Triglycerides, another type of "bad" blood fat, should be less than 150 mg/dL. Non-HDL cholesterol should be less than 130 mg/dL.

Many people take a drug to keep blood fats normal and reduce heart attack risk. And if you avoid foods high in animal fat/cholesterol, lose weight and exercise, even lower blood lipids are likely. Sometimes fasting triglycerides can go even lower to an ideal 100 mg/dL. Learn more about healthy foods from a "healthy heart" cookbook.

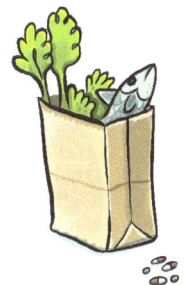

*If very high risk for heart attack, goals may be less than 70 mg/dL (LDL) and less than 100 mg/dL (non-HDL).

control high blood pressure

High blood pressure leads to damage of the lining of the arteries. This makes it easier for fatty buildup to occur and increases your risk of stroke. You can help control high blood pressure by making wise choices about foods, exercise, medicines and stress. An "ideal'" blood pressure at rest is less than 120/80. Ask your doctor about your target blood pressure goal.

exercise as prescribed

Exercise can help you to:

- lower LDLs (bad cholesterol) and triglycerides

- raise HDLs (good cholesterol)

- reach and keep a good weight

- reduce tension

- control blood pressure

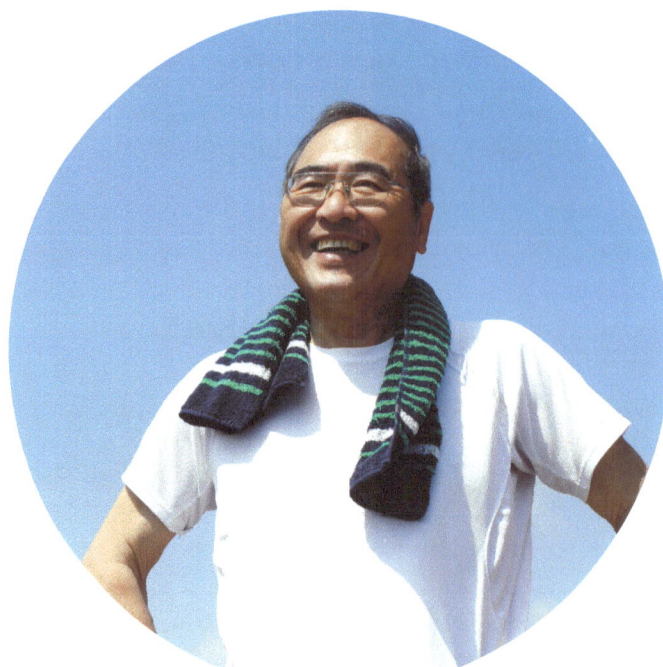

If your artery gets narrow again, exercise will help you notice the symptoms early and get help. Ask your doctor how much and what type of exercise is best for you.

lose weight if needed

Overweight people tend to have high blood cholesterol (and other blood fats) as well as a much higher rate of diabetes. Extra weight can make it harder to keep blood pressure under control. Ask your doctor what a good weight is for you.

learn to relax

Tension can make high blood pressure worse and may raise blood cholesterol and fat levels. Try to avoid people or things that upset you, and learn ways to relax.

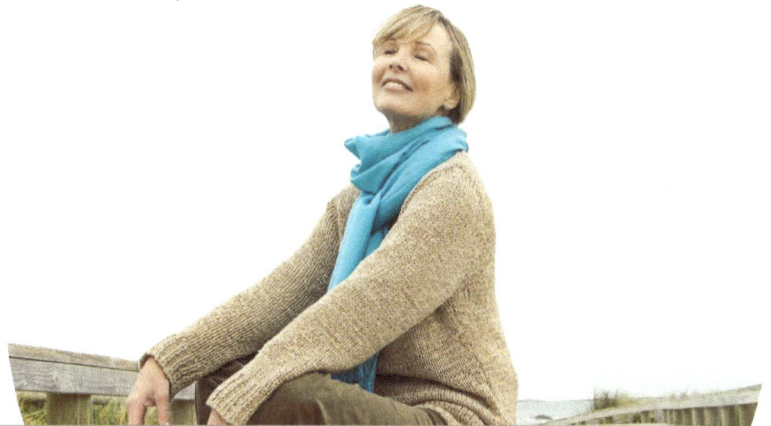

My Risk Factors and Goals												
	Now			3 month goal			6 month goal			1 year goal		
Smoking												
Cholesterol	HDL	LDL	Trig*	HDL	LDL	Trig*	HDL	LDL	Trig*	HDL	LDL	Trig*
Blood Pressure												
Exercise												
Weight												
Relaxation												

*Triglycerides

also...

People with **diabetes** are at greater risk for heart disease. This means your A.M. blood sugar should test between 70–130 mg/dL and 2 hours after starting a meal, you should test less than 180 mg/dL. Also, your glycated hemoglobin (A1C) should be less than 7%. AIC builds up during times of high blood sugar.

If **coronary heart disease occurs at an early age** (30–55) in your family, you need to work hard to control other risk factors that can lead to fatty buildup in your arteries.

Your doctor or nurse can help you find ways to change risk factors you may have. Your doctor may suggest a specialist, and there may be local groups that can help. Also, there are many self-help books to control the risk factors that lead to fatty buildup. Some of them are:

- **Exercise for Heart & Health**

- **It's Heartly Fare, makes sense out of fat, cholesterol and salt**

- **Blood Pressure Control**

- **Wake Up Call for Your Heart, 8 ways to reduce your risk for a heart attack**

- **Chill Out!...and control stress**

- **Balance Your Act, for adults with type 1 or type 2 diabetes**

- **The Sweet Truth about managing type 2 diabetes**

(Available from Pritchett & Hull. See the inside back cover for our toll-free phone number.)

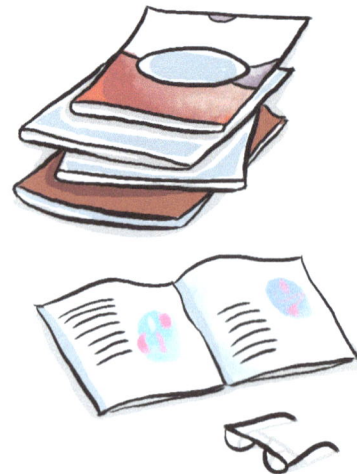

You can also visit the American Heart Association's website at www.heart.org for more information on preventing and controlling heart disease.

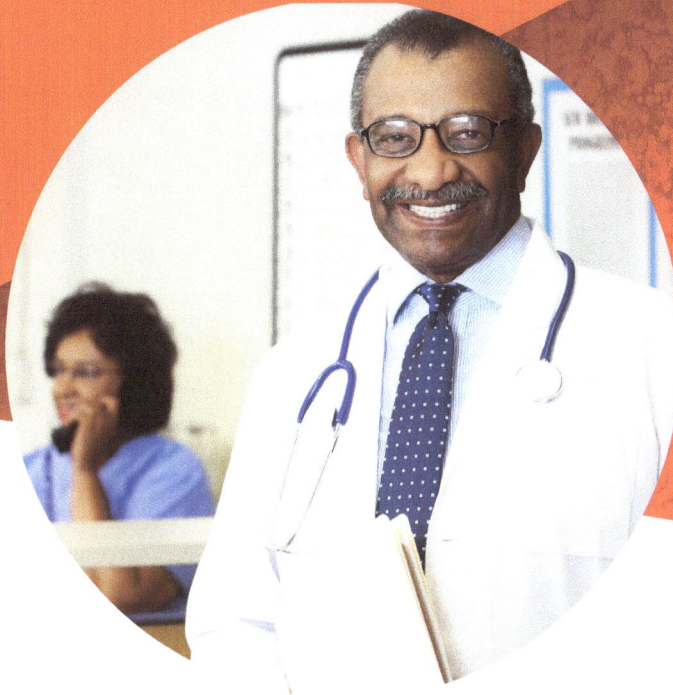

Some final words

Angioplasty has been done in leg arteries since 1969 and heart arteries since 1977. Some patients have no more trouble after angioplasty. But clots and buildup of smooth muscle cells or fatty plaque can occur.

Anti-clotting drugs are routine after angioplasty. **If a stent is used, anti-clotting drugs are vital.** Sometimes they are needed for weeks, but more often, for months or years. **Not taking the anti-clotting drugs could allow sudden clotting in the stent leading to heart attack or death.** Follow your doctor's advice about the length of time you need to take an anti-clotting drug.

Smooth muscle cells often build up on the artery wall after the "injury" of an angioplasty catheter or stent. This is called restenosis, but the drug-eluting stents (DES) and drug-coated balloons deliver a drug to discourage this over the coming months of healing. Anti-clotting drugs are still needed during the time a DES stent is delivering the drug and beyond.

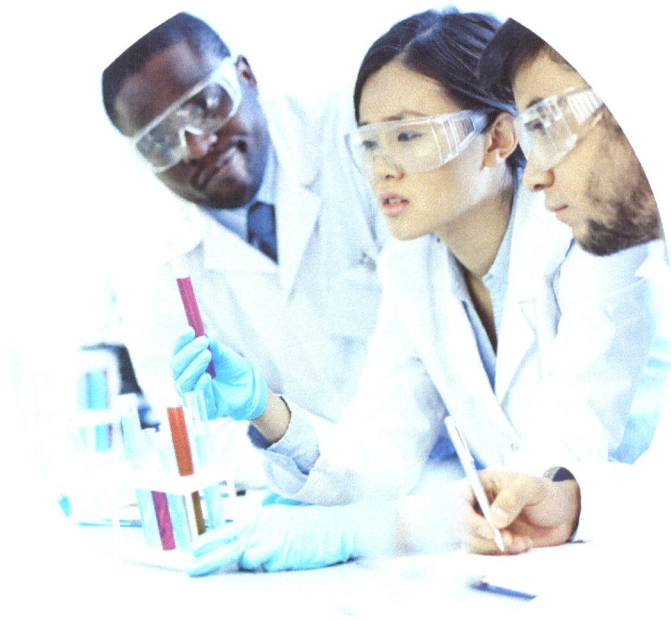

Some patients will need another angioplasty procedure or bypass surgery at some point. Scientists continue research in finding new ways to widen narrowed arteries and to prevent more artery narrowing.

Current research involves:

- gene testing/altering to:

  - correct high blood pressure, abnormal cholesterol levels and diabetes

  - determine anti-platelet drug dosage for prevention of blood clots and/or

  - detect coronary artery disease (peripheral gene expression)

- stem cells being injected into one or more heart arteries to encourage new arteries (angiogenesis)

- new imaging techniques in the heart arteries

- new stents (fully absorbable, designs suitable for tight narrowings and forks in arteries, and laser-drilled holes in stent struts for drug delivery)

- new drugs or combinations of drugs to prevent clotting

Notes

Order this book from :

PRITCHETT & HULL ASSOCIATES, INC.
3440 OAKCLIFF RD NE STE 126
ATLANTA GA 30340-3006

or call toll free: **800-241-4925**

Published and distributed by:
Pritchett & Hull Associates, Inc.

Printed in the U.S.A.

www.ingramcontent.com/pod-product-compliance
Lightning Source LLC
Chambersburg PA
CBHW060854270326
41934CB00002B/130